MINI HABITS
FOR
WEIGHT LOSS

Derrick White

TABLE OF CONTENTS

INTRODUCTION

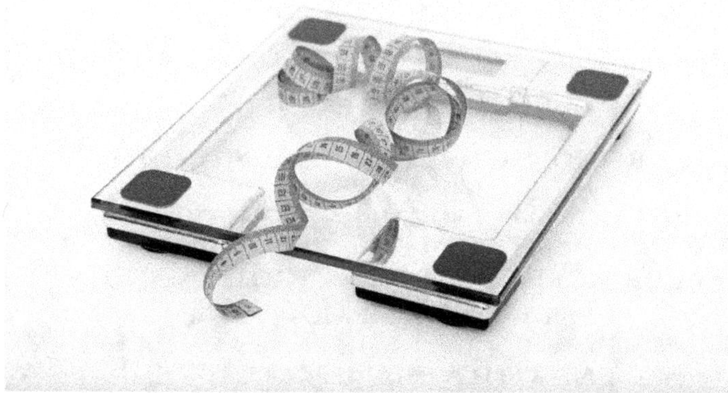

The increasing popularity of fad diets and green juice cleanses for weight loss has got us thinking that following a super strict diet and spending all our time in the gym are the only ways to lose weight. Fortunately for us, that isn't the case. Healthy and long-lasting weight loss is achievable only by making small but significant changes to our existing behavior. While fad diets have been advertised as the easiest way to drop a few pounds, they aren't sustainable, and you are bound to regain the lost weight and add extra pounds in the long run. The pattern of weight loss with fad diet; Angela adopts a new diet plan, the diet works, and she loses weight, she's excited and tell her friends about it, soon after she reverts to her normal life, she gains weight again and decide to start a new diet that has been trending for weeks, she starts a new diet, and repeats the process again.

Instead of taking your body through the unhealthy cycle of weight loss and regain, why not try these (?) mini habits not only to promote lasting and su-stainable weight loss but also improve your overall health. By developing healthy eating habits, you are not only losing weight, you'd also be losing the unhealthy habits and mindset that resulted in weight gain in the first instance. You are destroying the roots of unhealthy weight gain. While dieting ignites a big explosion that will burn out very quickly, mini habits ignite a small flame that overtime build a strong fire that will burn for a long time. Just like success, weight loss is a marathon, not a sprint!

TAKE 100% RESPONSIBILITY FOR YOUR HEALTH

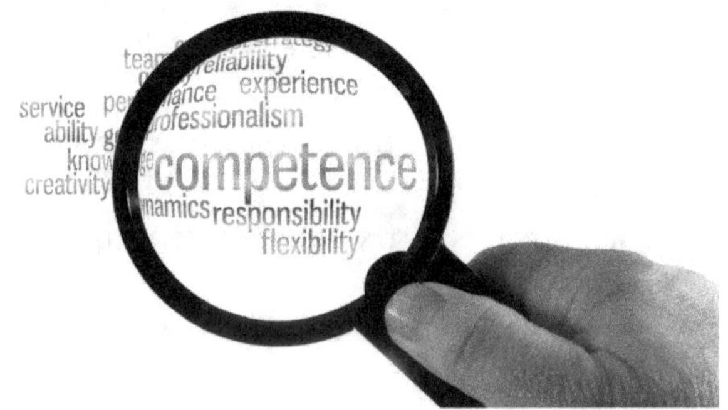

We have several systems in place today that has caused the death of self-responsibility. We buy and consume foods that are made by the food systems we have today. We buy all foods labeled "diet" for weight loss. These systems are taking away our control thus reducing our sense of responsibility. Don't get it wrong, there's absolutely nothing wrong with following a system that brings excellent results. But for systems that do not bring good results, it's up to us to leave and take 100% responsibility. Many overweight people today are overweight because that depend on food systems which actually promote obesity. Unfortunately, the weight loss and diets system that are meant to fix the problem are ineffective. What's left for you to do is to take 100% responsibility so you can lose weight and improve your overall health. This begs the question; how do we take back responsibility? The secret to take back responsibility is to start asking questions - will this diet actually help me or just give me false hope and short-term result? What about this smoothie, is it really 100% raw fruit with no artificial additive? What does food coloring do in my body? Is it even safe to eat it? These are all questions that most people do not care to ask, or do not have the time or knowledge to answer. But they are questions that matter, not only for long term weight loss but also to reduce the risk of diseases. Take full responsibility for your health regardless of your health status. Consider this - dieting makes people follow strict rules thus training them to give up their responsibility. This book will focus on healthy eating habits that will train you to take responsibility for your meal choices. If you want to succeed with weight loss, then you have to stop pressuring yourself to be at perfectly, make small but reasonable changes and take back responsibility. Decide from here on to take 100% responsibility for your weight and overall health. In the words of Sean Covey, "*We become what we repeatedly do.*"

#1. CUT DOWN ON SUGAR AND STARCH

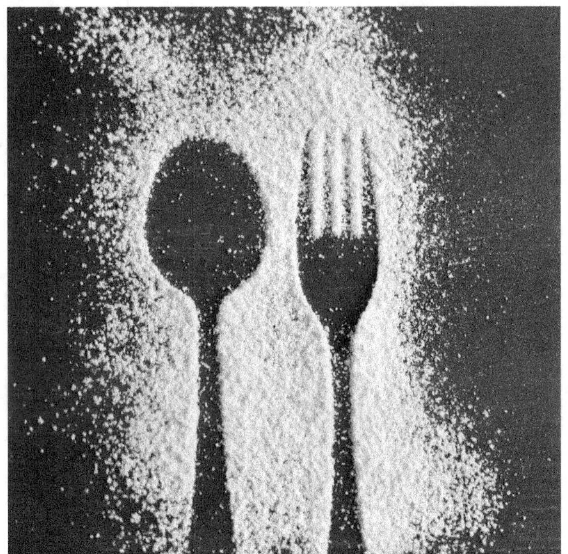

As far as sustainable weight loss is concerned, the most important step to take is to cut down, not eliminate, sugar and starch. Once you reduce the consumption of carbs (sugar and starch), your hunger levels also reduce thus making you eat less calories.

The effect this has on your body is, your body will burn stored fat for fuel not carbs.

More importantly, cutting down your carbs intake reduce your insulin levels and cause your kidneys to expel sodium and excess water from the body. So you can say goodbye to bloating and unnecessary water weight. When you cut down on sugar and starch, you can lose about 10 pounds in just one week. In simple words, cutting down on carbs intake is the secret to put weight loss on auto drive.

#2. INCLUDE MORE VEGETABLES, PROTEIN AND FAT IN YOUR MEAL

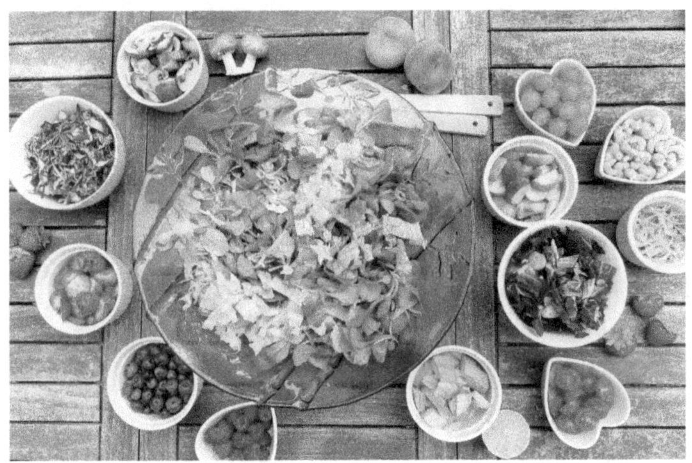

Your everyday meal should have a good mix of low carb vegetables, a protein and fat source. Planning your meals to include vegetables, protein and fat will automatically put your daily carb intake in the daily acceptable range of 20-25 grams. In addition to boosting your metabolism by 100 calories a day, daily intake of high protein foods also reduces cravings and obsession with food by 60%. You will also say goodbye to unhealthy late-night snacking.

Also, you can eat as much low carb vegetables as you want without eating more than the acceptable daily carbs intake. Including low carb vegetables in your meal will give you a perfect blend of fiber, vitamins, and minerals your body needs to be healthy.

Some vegetables to include in your meals.

- ❖ Broccoli

- ❖ Cauliflower

- ❖ Kale

- ❖ Tomatoes

- ❖ Spinach

*   Brussels sprouts

*   Cabbage

*   Cucumber

*   Lettuce

Protein

*   Fish and Seafood: Salmon, shrimp, trout, etc.

*   Meat: Lamb, pork, chicken, beef, etc.

*   Eggs: Whole eggs with the yolk are recommended.

Fats

*   Butter

*   Avocado oil

❖ Olive oil

❖ Coconut oil

#3. EAT WITH A SMALL PLATE

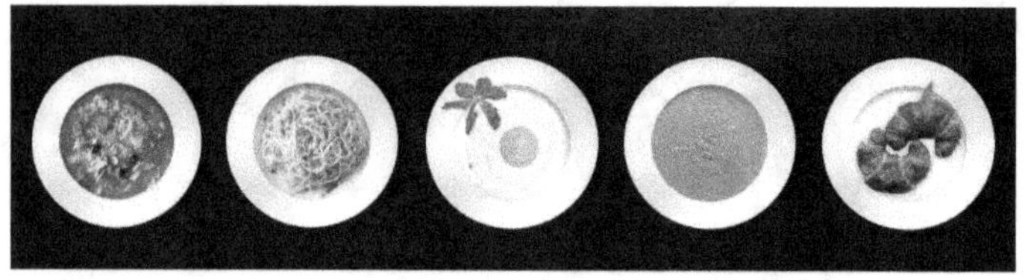

Research shows that the size of your plate affects your total calorie consumption. In essence, when you eat with a small plate, you eat fewer calories and on the flip side, when you eat with a big plate you automatically eat more calories. So it's safe to say that eating with a small plate helps us to control or reduce portion sizes which in turn causes low calorie consumption. You'd even be surprised that eating with a larger plate doesn't make you fully satisfied. In a recent research, participants who ate from a larger plate do not report experiencing higher level of satiety at the end of the meal. In other words, when we eat with a larger plate and serve a large portion of food, we tend to ignore satiety signals.

A recent study linked obesity with large portion sizes. In other words, large portion sizes contribute to the lifestyle disease that is prevalent across the world.

#4. PRACTICE MINDFUL EATING

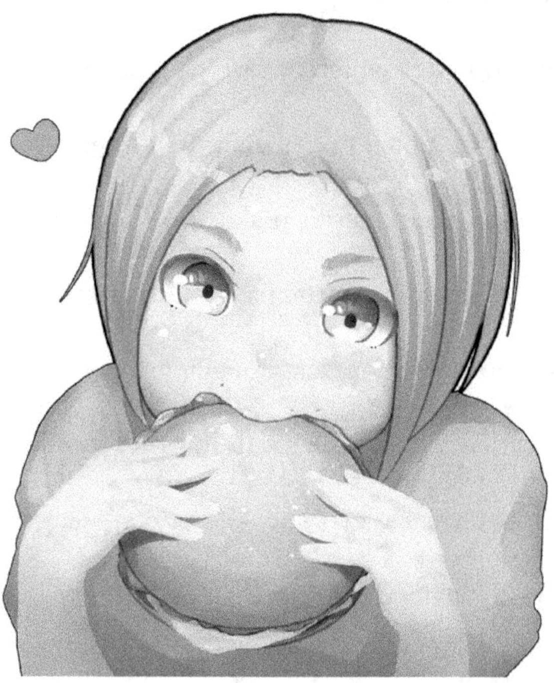

When it comes to long term weight loss, it's necessary to get yourself familiar with your hunger and fullness cues. Healthy eating and sustainable weight loss can be achieved only when you know the signals your body sends when you are hungry and when you are full. This begs the question, what's mindful eating?

Mindful eating is a method of eating that promotes your awareness while eating. While you are focusing on your meal, you are also looking out for signals to indicate that you are full. Health experts advise mindful eating as it has significant effects on eating behaviors and weight loss.

#5. CULTIVATE THE HABIT OF CHEWING GUM

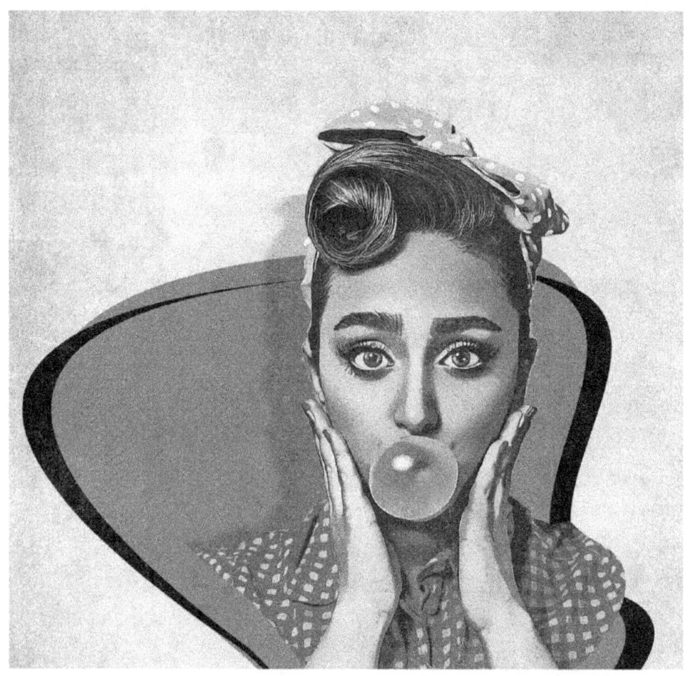

If you don't enjoy chewing gum, you may need to consider chewing gum as an alternative to snacking.

Whenever you feel the urge to snack on unhealthy foods, get your gum from your purse and chew.

Chewing gum can send false signals to your brain and stomach that it's getting real food. More importantly, the flavor of the gum stimulates the release of saliva in the mouth which in turn reduces appetite. Likewise, the enzymes in the saliva breaks down fat and starch in the body.

#6. BRUSH YOUR TEETH AFTER EACH MEAL

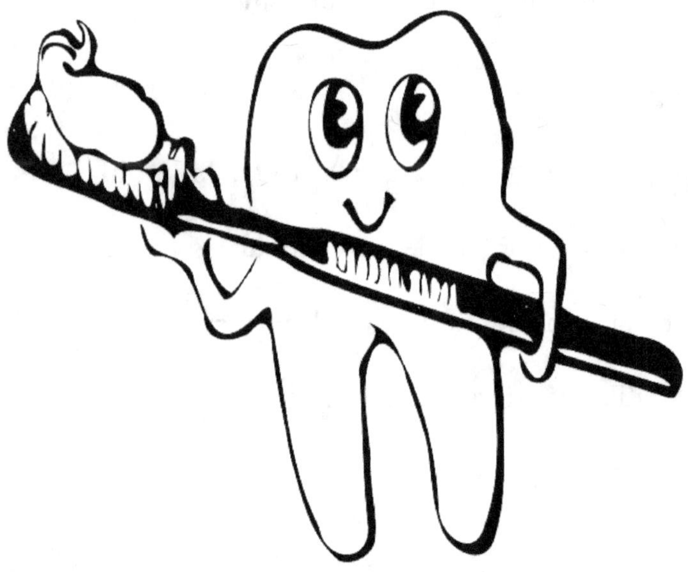

Health experts advise brushing our teeth after each

meal, not only to keep the teeth healthy and strong

but also to reduce the urge to snack after each meal.

There are people who do not like eating after brushing because they feel an awkward taste in their mouth. If you are one of those people, then you should take advantage of it. Make a simple habit of brushing after each meal so you don't snack in between your meals. A mouthwash is a good alternative to brushing.

#7. NO TV WHILE EATING

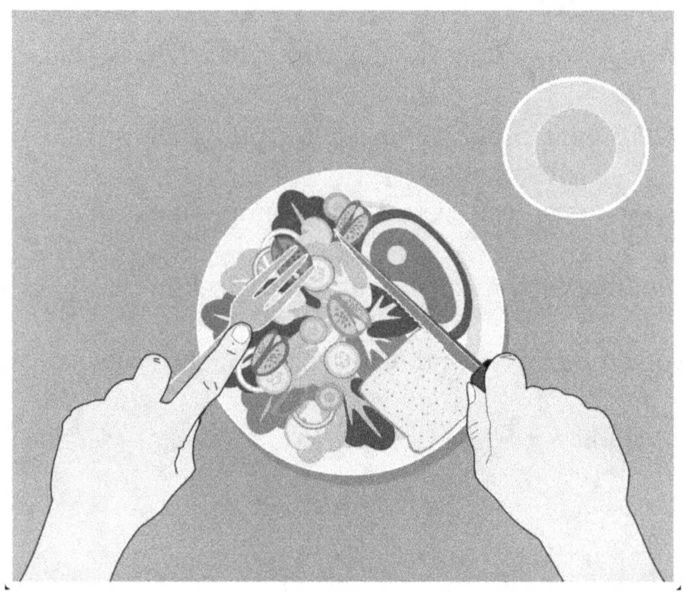

Practicing mindful eating can be difficult when you
are watching TV, checking Facebook for notificati-
ons or scrolling through Instagram feeds when you
are eating. You may think that doing other things

while you are eating will make you eat less but in reality; you will actually eat more than necessary.

Giving in to distractions while eating doesn't only affect the current meal, it also makes you eat more than needed in other meals. When possible, get rid of all distractions and focus on your meal.

#8. DRINK WATER 24/7

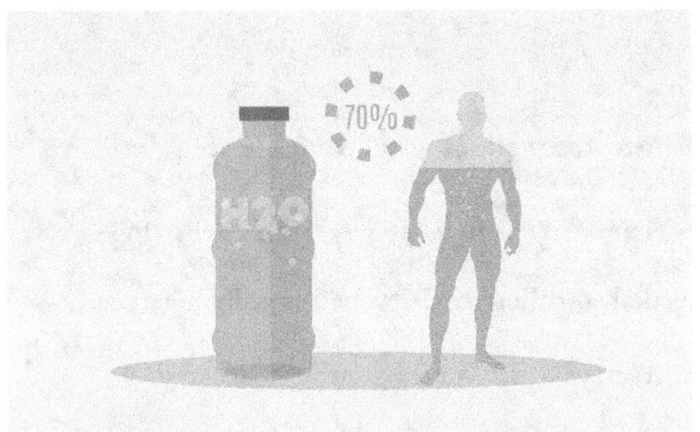

Since high school, we have learnt the importance of water in the body. Why not consider drinking water before your meals to promote fullness? Research shows that drinking water before meals increase weight loss by 44% in a period of three months.

Even though the body is a brilliant machine, slip-ups are entirely avoidable. Sometimes what you think is hunger may not be hunger for food but water. That hunger can make you snack on unhealthy foods when all your body wants is just water. Perhaps you aren't a fan of plain water. You can infuse fruits in your water to encourage drinking more water.

#9. SQUEEZE IN SOME EXERCISE

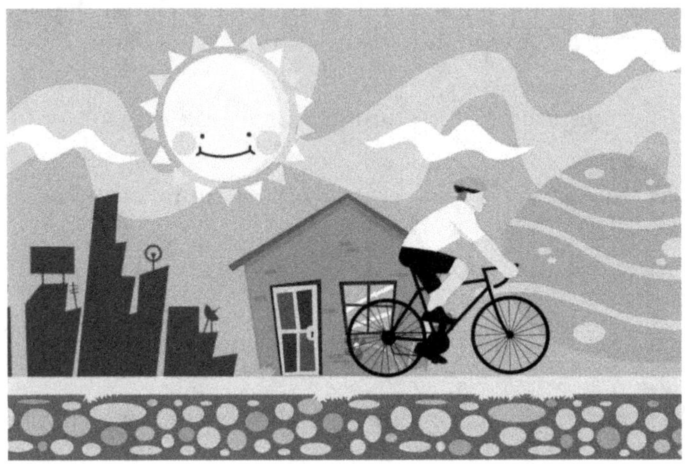

Engaging in physical activity in the morning helps to promote weight loss. As far as long-term weight loss is concerned, you cannot rule out physical activity.

Engaging in physical activity in the morning helps to regulate your blood sugar level thus preventing low blood sugar that can cause negative symptoms which includes excessive hunger.

If you are unable to exercise in the morning, you can incorporate physical activity in your daily routine. Take the stairs instead of the elevator, walk around the block, walk your dog to the park, take a 30-minute brisk walk in the evening.

#10. HAVE A STRESS OUTLET THAT'S NOT FOOD

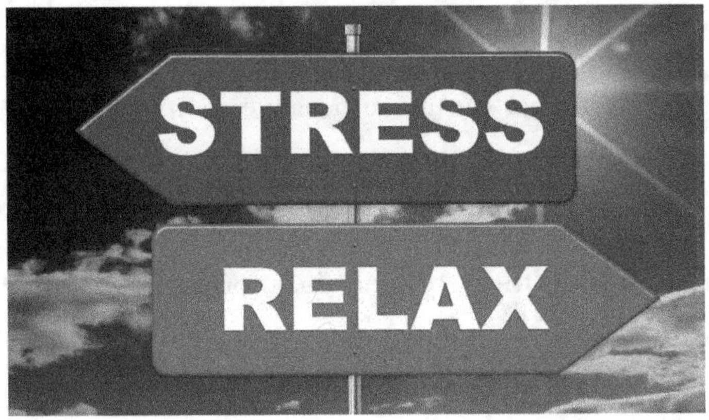

Have a stress outlet different from food - a study conducted by professors at the University of Alabama found that people who eat more as a response to emotional stress are thirteen times more likely to develop obesity and be overweight.

Whenever you are emotionally stressed or going through a difficult day and you have the urge to eat as a response to the stress, drink a tall glass of infused water instead, chew a piece of gum or take a walk around the block.

Have a stress outlet that's not good and you will stop yourself from excessive eating and overloading on calories.

CONCLUSION

In the words of Sean Covey, we become what we repeatedly do. Decide now to unlearn old habits and learn new healthy eating habits that will put your weight loss on autopilot.

As you practice the mini habits for weight loss discussed in this book, you will begin to create a healthy environment in your mind and body, which will encourage weight loss. Achieving your weight loss and body goals is now within your reach - decide from here on to take full responsibility for your body, weight, and overall health.

Choose to be healthy!

Images

Scale Diet Fat - Free photo on Pixabay

Competence Experience Hand - Free photo on Pixabay

Spoon Fork Cutlery Icing - Free photo on Pixabay

Salad Fruits Berries - Free photo on Pixabay

Food Dishes Meal - Free photo on Pixabay

Moe Rice Eat - Free image on Pixabay

Woman Female Retro - Free image on Pixabay

Toothbrush Brush Hygiene - Free vector graphic on Pixabay

Food Healthy Hands - Free vector graphic on Pixabay

Water Drink Body - Free vector graphic on Pixabay

Park City Bicycle - Free image on Pixabay

Stress Relaxation Relax - Free image on Pixabay

www.ingramcontent.com/pod-product-compliance
Lightning Source LLC
Chambersburg PA
CBHW050757250726
48662CB00005B/2271